NICKI JEFFERY

Precious Michelle

A Sister Reminisces a Life Lost to Suicide

Foreword

'Precious Michelle' is a celebration of the incredible life of a beautiful Christian woman. We are not defined by the way we die. Our weakest moments, our times of illness, and our scars are part of our human condition. We are all broken. But we have a Saviour.

Our Saviour Jesus holds us in our every moment. He never leaves us. Not even for a millisecond. Not even when we despair of life. And especially in our seasons of pain.

* * *

I venture down the beach and I think of you splashing in the waves, laughing and smiling. Racing along the sand when we were kids, your cap in your hand and hair swept back by the wind. Snapshots in time.

I start my motorbike and button up your jacket—one of your articles of clothing I keep to wear and remember you. The revs remind me of countless seasons mustering sheep together. We'd idle along behind the flock and to the side. Then we'd pause and play 'paper, scissors, rock' to keep us entertained.

I sing a worship song and raise my eyes heavenward. You're there beside me, melodies flowing from your lips and heart to your King. And heaven is smiling at the passion on your face.

I watch butter melt in my banquet frypan and pour beaten eggs in. As they bubble and sizzle, I think of you. Fried rice was your favourite meal. With each mouthful I reflect on meals shared and thanks given.

Life is not the same without you. When you appear in my dreams and you're alive and well; my heart rejoices. You are with me again, at least for a moment.

I have been bereaved by suicide, and I've felt suicidal. I'm still here to tell the story. One of the reasons I'm here is Michelle.

But this is not my story. It's the story of a warrior in the Kingdom of heaven. A fun-loving, dream-chasing daughter of the Most High God. Precious Michelle.

While she is no longer with us, Michelle was a writer. The journal entries interwoven throughout this book are her story and through them, you will hear her heart and her voice.

* * *

To watch the eight minute documentary, 'Precious Michelle', made by the Mid North Coast Mental Health Integrated Multimedia team ~

https://www.nickijeffery.com/precious-michelle/

Preface

My depression has worried me this time. I haven't had particular suicidal thoughts (as in a plan) but my mind has definitely been wandering into that territory, God help me. I do just want the pain and discomfort to end so badly.[1]

It was Friday when Mum phoned me, sounding out of breath.

'Michelle's not coping. She's not sleeping or eating, and she's having trouble making decisions. I'm sorry, Nicki. We won't be coming over this weekend. I've got to stay here and look after your sister.'

It was Mother's Day in Australia, Sunday 14th May, when Michelle presented at emergency at her local hospital. Four hospitals and 11 days later, Michelle was dead.[2]

Acknowledgement

Precious Michelle rose

The rose behind Michelle's face on the book cover is called 'Precious Michelle'. My beautiful friend, Natasha, was sad to hear the news of my sister's passing. She knew Michelle personally and as she was praying one day, she heard the words 'Precious Michelle' over and over in her heart. She decided to do a Google search. Natasha discovered that 'Precious Michelle' is a rose. Knowing that roses were Michelle's favourite flowers, she ordered 'Precious Michelle' rose plants and sent one to my parents, and one to me. The photo on the book cover is a rose that bloomed from this plant.

In addition, the Mid North Coast Mental Health Integrated Multimedia team named their documentary 'Precious Michelle'.

A heartfelt thank you to Natasha and to the team.

One

Michelle the Sister

Out of the shadows of two older sisters, Michelle Louise Williams the actress emerged. She loved to sing and dance and was often melodramatic. She had a way with words and was always penning beautiful, heartfelt cards and letters to friends and family. She was good at drawing. Good at cross country running. She played a nice game of tennis, loved motorbike riding and water-skied on a single ski.

Dad and Grandad were share farmers and graziers on adjoining farms in the central west slopes and plains of New South Wales, Australia. Mum and Grandma were housewives and both stayed home to raise their children and support their men on the land.

A few times every summer, we took our ski boat to Gum Bend Lake near Condobolin for a day of water-skiing, a barbecue lunch, and bags of mixed lollies from the kiosk, then choc-coated ice-creams from the corner store on our way home to the farm.

When Lucinda was born, there were four girls: Kelly, Nicole, Michelle and Lucinda. The two youngest became known as 'the little ones'. The middle two girls were like two peas in a pod. No sons, but essentially four tomboys growing up on a sheep and wheat farm.

Sometimes I wonder why Michelle and I got along so famously. Was it our opposite personalities? Michelle was wise and discerning, while I am a bit gullible and tend to speak before I think. Michelle was moody and stubborn, while I am optimistic and somewhat selfish.

Was it that we had so much time to play together as kids? Was it that I was a dreamer and Michelle a realist? While share-driving in North America and camping along the way, my thoughts were on the manuscript I was writing, while Michelle thought through our stops. While I dreamed up Jay and Lana's romance, Michelle pointed out the fact that we didn't have boyfriends and our own love lives were likely to remain absent whilst we travelled.

Here are the words Michelle penned in my twenty-first autograph book:

I can't believe you're 21! Life seems to move so quickly it only seems like yesterday that we were climbing trees and in your case stopping to pick the paper flowers. You have a tremendous ability to colour the world brightly and only see the good in things and people. As a realist and I stress that word, I will never be that way. I guess that's why we get along so well. I'm chained to your ankle so when you drift too high in your fantasy world I can pull you down to reality. I can't imagine a better sister or friend.

We've been through a lot together and have a lot more to get through together.
There's nothing quite like a solid friendship. We were sisters and best friends—'best sisters'. If a soul mate exists for us in terms of friendship, that's what we were to each other.

One warm evening when I was about twelve years old, Mum was not happy with me.

I was halfway across the paddock heading for the dam, tears filling my eyes. I had to get away.

Michelle ran after me. 'Hey, Nic!'

We sat panting on the dam bank, side by side.

'My life is ruined.' I hung my head and used my fingernail to loosen the jagged stones. I lifted my gaze, tears mingling with sweat on my red cheeks. 'My friend had a birthday party and I didn't want to go. Now Mum's talking to her mum on the phone. She's trying to explain why I wouldn't go. And I've just run off, refusing to talk to my only three friends. I can't go back to school on Monday. My life is over.'

Weekends were my time on the farm with my family. Weekdays, Kelly and I boarded with a family in town so we could attend the Christian school when I was in year seven. I didn't know it then, but I was anxious and being home on the farm was my safe place.

Michelle's eyes were brimming with empathy and understanding. She dug her chin into her shoulder and sighed. 'I've lost my library book and now I'm going to have to pay for it. That's all my pocket money gone for the rest of the year!'

I put my arm around my sister. Michelle was never a big hugger, but she relaxed a little and took a deep breath.

We stood and tried our best to skim stones over the surface of the dam.

Michelle and I shared a bedroom for a while. You could tell whose side was whose. Michelle's wardrobe contained folded clothes and the doors were shut. Her books and toys were squared away. My cupboard bulged with clothes and papers. The doors were always opened and the carpet was covered in creative projects. But somehow it worked.

Saturday mornings were always the same when we were kids. Michelle and I ran to the lounge room dragging our pink and purple doonas behind us. We turned the TV on to Prime at seven am for 'Saturday Disney'[3]. We took a lounge each and lay down in cosy comfort, enjoying our favourite American kids' shows— 'Duck Tales', 'TailSpin', 'Saved by the Bell'[4].

It's no wonder we always dreamed of travelling to the USA. I completed three years of full-time teaching while Michelle completed her first university degree in Early Childhood education. No boyfriends, no mortgages, no children—we were free to travel. Michelle discovered Work Canada—twelve-month working holiday visas to Canada that needed to be obtained before we turned thirty-one. We thought we would teach in the USA, but that seemed a bit complex to achieve. Working and travelling in Canada, with the option of travelling for a few months in the USA was appealing. We did it! It was the trip of a lifetime.

I met Michelle at Toronto airport after spending three months in the States as a summer camp counsellor. We worked in Ontario, then flew to Vancouver. We found jobs at Big White Ski Resort near Kelowna. Then to escape the icy conditions, we flew to Los Angeles and across to the Hawaiian Islands. Back on the east coast of the USA, we bought a car thanks to Dad's generosity, and we drove to Las Vegas and the Grand Canyon before heading back up to Canada, then right across the bottom of the nation to Prince Edward Island in the east. We worked and travelled. We also spent time in Florida before returning home to Australia.

Flying to the west coast of Canada without jobs lined up was a real test of our faith and our trust in God to provide. We arrived in Kelowna, British Columbia, the day before Big White Ski Resort held its Hospitality Job Fair. Unfortunately, the shuttle bus up the mountain was all booked. Would anyone cancel in the morning? Yes! Two guys decided to go shopping instead and my sister and I were hired and worked at the ski resort for four months.

Kind-hearted people took us in over and over again as we journeyed. After leaving Severn Lodge in Ontario for the second time, we headed to Ottawa, having lunch with a lady along the way. She provided us with a contact and two nights' accommodation with her friends. These French Canadians were the loveliest Christian family and the best hosts we ever had.

Not only were they excellent conversationalists, but they provided big breakfasts of pastries, fruit, yoghurt, juice and cereals, as well as thinking to give us cold bottles of water for the day. We were welcomed in as members of their family.

Overseas, Michelle and I had a kind of joint identity as 'the sisters'. And back home, Michelle had long been in my shadow—at school, then university. But in our final church in Canada, the pastor's wife prophesied over us. She said, 'You are sisters, not overshadowed by each other. You are individuals in God's sight with separate callings.'

We took sister bushwalks to the waterhole at the base of a big hill on our parents' new farm. (They moved to another regional area when we were about to travel to Canada.) Some days the water flowed, but most times it trickled over the rocks. In the afternoon shadows, sitting amongst pine trees and sheep droppings, we shared our hearts.

The January after Michelle and I returned from overseas, Lucinda joined us at the waterhole. We reflected on our lives and the various decisions we had to make. We prayed for godly wisdom for Lucinda as she was considering studying veterinary science at university in Wagga Wagga, and direction for Michelle since she was thinking of heading there too. We prayed for God to prepare my heart and mind for YWAM (Youth With A Mission) in Brisbane.

Our lives headed in different directions after that. I lived with our parents on their new farm until I went to YWAM in Brisbane, and Michelle headed down to Wagga Wagga to make her home with Lucinda for a few years.

When we did end up back in town together, I was married and expecting a baby.

Life wasn't the same for the sisters anymore. Not only did my marriage trigger a divide between us but moving to the coast and suffering post-natal depression tested our relationship.

Like all of the members of my biological family, Michelle wanted to see me flourish. She began to view my husband with suspicion, concluding that he might be responsible for my battle with mental illness. Was he abusive in some way? Michelle shared her views with me when I was at my most vulnerable, and this triggered a bigger divide that took years to rectify.

Relationships are messy, even between best sisters. But Michelle's heart was always to see me well and thriving. And years later, my husband initiated a hard conversation with my sister. They repaired their connection. And when my sons were five and three, she and I had our own 'sister weekend' at the Gold Coast. The relationship was mended and we were back. The lines of communication opened. Hearts poured out. Hugs and tears. The Michelle I had always known and loved came rushing back into my life like a long-lost friend.

Michelle always wrote lovely birthday cards to me. Here's a snippet from one of them:

I pray that you always know how deeply loved you are by me. We've spent most of our lives together exploring the world and our own backyards. My prayer is that you also know how much of a treasure you are to God and that you see yourself as He sees you. Lots of love, Michelle.

Two

Michelle the Tomboy

Chocolate brown eyes under a navy cap sparkled with a hint of mischief. Long, slender fingers gripped motor-bike handles as a leg poised ready to kick-start the 250. That cheeky smile emerged with the roar of the engine. And she was gone, a puff of red dust following the farm girl up the paddock.

The year of Michelle's rural traineeship cemented her love of farming and all things 'Dad'.

'We're going to check on the sheep in the 180,' Dad said over breakfast, his spoon chinking the sides of his Weetbix bowl. 'Then I've got to hoe out the Bathurst burrs in the yabby dam paddock.'

Michelle nodded, heaving the basket of wet washing onto the table. 'I'll cook fish fingers and chips for lunch again; our favourite.' She winked and cackled—her easy laugh.

Everyone who heard it knew it was Michelle; that contagious laugh that made you smile.

Michelle hung the washing out to dry, shirts flapping in the breeze. Then she pulled on her overalls and gumboots to join Dad. She treasured this time.

It was nice for her not to be living in town anymore. When Mum's father passed away, our mother had the opportunity to move into his house in town. She did this, taking Michelle, Lucinda and me with her for our schooling during the week, then home to the farm on weekends. Three years later, Mum and Lucinda were still in town to finish off Lucinda's schooling. That meant Dad and Michelle were always together working on the farm during her gap year.

Michelle was pleased to be free of high school. At pre-school age, she had gone everywhere with Dad. There was no prying her away. No daycare, no one-day-a-week of pre-school for her. She started 'big' school on day one. None of this education before kindergarten business. Farm life was education.

For Michelle, it was full circle taking a year off after high school. Back to the land. Back to the bush. She often dashed through the bush with the dogs, leaping over logs and crackling dry leaves with each step, balancing on fallen tree trunks as rabbits darted down burrows and grey kangaroos jumped between the ironbark trees.

At home, Michelle would sit on the veranda spitting seeds from the mandarin she'd picked from the tree in the garden. She knew where to find her favourite fruits if dinner wasn't to her liking Then she might sit in the tree or atop the gate near the rainwater tank to eat.

As a kid, she'd loved climbing trees and riding the branches like they were horses. She'd throw her head back and laugh, flicking imaginary reins and patting her stallion on his neck. She was brave on the backs of real horses too. Michelle was the only one of the girls in our family to spend much time riding the neighbour's horses. We were a motorbike family and Dad wasn't into horses. She was persistent in learning to ride. And one year on a family holiday down at Lakes Entrance in Victoria, she revelled in a trail ride we took through the beautiful forest. Lucinda and I were beginners at riding, but Michelle had a knack for trotting and cantering.

December 1998

My ambition is to live by the beach near Nicki on a small farm and to have horses.

Michelle loved Beauty, her black and white cat. She cuddled kittens and puppies, nursed lambs, and once tried to help a mother mouse feed her eight babies up in the chook yard! Jumping over stinging nettles, Michelle tended to the animals. Farm life delighted her.

She loved driving the orange Suzuki. Weekday mornings at 7:20 am, three sisters ran out to the manual vehicle, fighting over who would drive to the bus stop that day. Whoever didn't drive and had the passenger seat would be opening and closing all the gates.

'I got all the gates yesterday!' I whined.

'The last one out of the house has to get the gates.' Michelle said, retying her black hair band.

'I'm driving,' Kelly declared, taking the wheel.

And off we motored up the red dirt road, dodging potholes because we knew where each one was. Past the haystack with the surrounding gum trees and swooping magpies in Spring. By the corner of a paddock where Kelly had once found a dead fox. And up the lane towards Grandad and Grandma's house. They would always be waiting on the veranda to wave to their grandchildren driving past.

Michelle learnt to drive trucks and tractors. When ploughing the paddocks, she knew to look through the rear-view mirror and raise the plough as she curved around kurrajong trees. That way the tree roots stayed underground, nourishing the trunk. The red puffs of dust lingered behind, like clouds from the stomping feet of giants.

She could reverse the wheat-filled dump truck up to the silo, stopping at the strategically positioned piece of wood. She pull-started the auger with a rope and watched the wheat granules shake up the cylinder into their destination. Other days, she hoisted heavy bags of wheat and oats to feed the sheep.

Each Christmas our many cousins, aunts and uncles came 'home' to our farm to spend time with Grandad and Grandma and their country cousins. There were twin aunties: Libby and Mary-Anne, along with their husbands and children: Uncle John and his wife and two kids, and Aunty Jean and her husband and three kids.

After present giving, we ran outside to play around the sheds and silos, surrounded by clucking chooks and loyal kelpies. Altogether there were 16 cousins picking and throwing little squishy paddy melons around the orchard. Handball, tips, cricket, board games and table tennis kept us busy, and we chatted and laughed it up until lunchtime.

A delicious spread of roast turkey, ham on the bone, jellied salads, buttery mashed potato, tomato and onion topped with sugar, and homemade mayonnaise cluttered the table. Dad said grace and we loaded our plates and found a spot to sit out on the splintery veranda or on the lounges. We all made room for dessert because Grandma was the most amazing cook. Plum pudding, a myriad of jellies, pavlova, ice-cream, fruit cake and egg custard tantalised our taste buds.

'Let's play barbie dolls,' one of our cousins would say. Michelle played a little, but much preferred running around outside with her older sisters and cousins.

A favourite game was playing 'community' on the tennis court. Our oldest kelpie, Mack, loved it when we played, as he would dash from side to side outside the fence with every shot. He wore a nice little track beside the clay court. We all jumped on—probably six or so a side. We hit the ball to one another, sitting it out when we missed a volley or messed up the shot. When an entire team was out, we mixed up the players and began again. Then we dove into our above ground swimming pool to cool off and do backflips and somersaults.

December 2005

I walked over to the Lucerne and had a couple of shots. Later Dad came on his four wheeler and he rode while I sat on the back and shot at the rabbits. It was awesome! He took me for a ride on his Harley-Davidson as well. I have such special memories with Dad. I just want to treasure them all in my heart.

It wouldn't be long before Michelle the tomboy would gain a new identity in the big, wide world. A career or two, a degree or two, a life far removed from the safety of the farm in the central west slopes and plains. She would become an early childhood teacher and a social worker, her heart taking her to places she needed to go.

Three

Michelle the Traveller

I wrote the following piece for Faithwriters weekly writing challenge whilst Michelle was alive. The topic was 'Traveller'. At Michelle's funeral, I read this alongside Dad, who also gave a eulogy.

The pretty brunette exhales atop the mountain range. Skinny fingers sling her backpack down in the snow. Brown eyes shine as she beholds the splendid view. She laughs and lifts her hands to heaven.

My sister was a single, thirty-something-year-old world traveller, who was, by day, a child protection counsellor. A few weeks a year, wanderlust was her passion.

Michelle was twenty-three when she took her first overseas trip from native Australia to Canada.

She started in Toronto, Ontario, and spent twelve months on a working holiday visa in the States and North America.

Michelle caught the travel bug.

Her adventures took her from safari in Africa to the beauty of Europe and the wilds of the Amazon jungle.

On social media she posted, *Just returned from the holiday of a lifetime! The world is an amazing place.*

With a heart for kids, particularly troubled youths, she spent time working in a juvenile detention centre. Her first university degree was in early childhood teaching, her second social work.

She had a beautiful heart, crafted by her heavenly Father. Since the age of nine, she had called Jesus Lord. Michelle always attended church, served on various teams, led Bible studies and drew her friends into fellowship. She was pure in body and spirit. A true princess—daughter of the King.

For her first mission trip, Michelle worked in Watoto Baby Home in Kampala, Uganda's capital city. She was assigned to the 'Hippo Room', caring for twelve-month-old babies. The little boys and girls came from hospitals where mothers gave birth and left, or were brought in off the streets and from garbage dumps by police. Many had HIV.

Photos of Michelle from this time show my sister sitting down on the ground, and half a dozen babies lying on her drinking milk from bottles. Michelle's smile is radiant. I think God smiles when He thinks of that time.

Two years before Michelle passed away, she spent five weeks in South America. On her single wage and with a house mortgage, she sponsored five children. She visited three on her trip—Lisandro in San Salvador, Juan in Managua and Pedro in Guayaquil. They were blessed during this time with her presence, and the Nike soccer balls she gave them. Not to mention the finances and letters she sent over the years. They are her spiritual sons.

Picture a beautiful woman with a listening ear and wise counsel, who was a thoughtful, compassionate friend and then hear her lovely soprano singing voice worshipping God. She sounded like a mighty intercessor praying for her clients.

Watch as she jumps out of a plane, skydiving over an aqua ocean, plummeting down raging rapids in a white water raft, then trekking through forests, perspiration beading under her cap.

The pretty brunette exhales atop the mountain range. Skinny fingers sling her backpack down in the snow. Brown eyes shine as she beholds the splendid view. She laughs and lifts her hands to heaven.

'Only ask, and I will give you the nations as your inheritance, the whole earth as your possession.'[5]

Over thirteen years, Michelle travelled to five continents, experiencing their beauty and diversity and making many new friends. Travel for her represented new opportunities. She loved seeing different places. To have a holiday and to travel overseas helped refresh her for the hard work in child protection she did back in Australia, and it was a reprieve from any personal issues she was dealing with.

December 2009

The trip changed my life completely! I fell in love with the gorgeous babies at Baby Watoto, especially my 'son' Freddy and the people of Uganda.

Michelle felt at her best in nature. She could climb a mountain, snorkel off islands, taste new cuisine. Plummet down rapids, enjoy a roaring campfire, marvel at a waterfall.

January 2009

The boat ride in Uganda was absolutely spectacular! I went upstairs onto the viewing platform and saw thousands of hippos, crocodiles, elephants, warthogs, birds, antelope, lizards and more. We arrived at the falls a few hours later which were amazing.

Daring, adventurous, winsome Michelle was at home on the dusty red trails surrounding Uluru, bungee jumping from a gorge or patting lion cubs in an East African game park. She had the drive and the confidence to take journeys with Jesus.

June 2004

Uluru and Kata Tjuta have been absolutely breathtaking. The sacred sites are wondrous and I like to picture where the Anangu people camped and taught their children; such a beautiful culture.

It felt like a water ride at a theme park as we propelled down the rapids. In a flurry of bubbles, we paddled frantically, with every dip of our inflatable raft. The river flowed down a chasm about ten metres wide, rocks protruding through the froth. The roar of the water was broken only by the periodic shouts of our guide.

In Australia, Michelle and me had both skydived, parasailed and gone on the scariest roller coasters theme parks could offer us. We had always wanted to add white-water rafting to our list of extreme sports conquered. Our weekend white-water rafting was the extreme getaway for counsellors from the Ontario spring camp.

Rafting reminded me that the waves in the stormy sea of life are perilous. Sharp rocks beneath the surface threaten to rip us apart if we don't stay in the raft with Jesus.[6]

There were times when Michelle struggled with fears and bouts of depression, but she kept these to herself and revelled in her freedom.

Michelle's journals are full of her thoughts on the places she ventured to, but they also contain writing on the people she met—friendships made, struggles they faced, her heart for them.

Her travels were about exploring and connecting. Michelle had a way of relating with others allowing each soul to share as she listened reflectively. Her passion for justice shone through her eyes and came through her carefully chosen words.

March 2015

God is giving my life purpose far greater than I could have imagined.

My trip to Canada, the USA and the Hawaiian Islands with Michelle was a highlight of my twenties. I expected to meet and marry the man of my dreams in my early twenties, and I spent many nights upset and crying about my perpetual single situation. To be having adventures in new places away from the world of my coupled friends, was a reprieve. I'm so glad we took the plunge and travelled together while we were able to. We will never have the chance to fulfil our pinkie promise to take our husbands and children back to Disneyworld in Florida, but Michelle met my family and we look forward to being with her in heaven, which will be so much better than Disneyworld!

Two dear friends I met overseas wrote these emails when we returned home:

'It was awesome knowing you and I'm glad you and Michelle had an awesome, God-filled adventure.'

'What an impact the 'Williams sisters' have made in the lives they have touched. It is amazing how God divinely planned your time with us and with all your other contacts this past year. I am so thankful to have the closeness with you both.'

February 2009

The adventure is over but it's great to be home.

Four

Michelle the Friend

'Let's go, guys!' Michelle spun around, reflected light dancing from her dangly earrings.

The dorm common room was abuzz with the latest Top 40 songs. Half-finished alcoholic drinks sat on tables and benchtops. University students stood in small groups, some laughing and telling stories, others were swaying to the beat.

'You ready to get on the hard stuff?' a dorm mate joked, swishing Michelle's glass of plain lemonade.

Michelle pulled a face, 'Yeah, right. You know I just want to dance.'

Dressed in black pants and shimmery silver top, her petite figure was a head-turner. Her smile could light up the uni bar and her laugh could brighten any dark corner. Her brunette hair fell to her shoulders, straight and styled. She walked with an extra bounce in her step.

Thursday nights at the uni bar were the highlight of each week. And Michelle was in her element. Bands visiting the university played covers, then DJ music filled their breaks. Michelle sang and danced the night away.

December 2003

I think I'm going to miss the social aspect of university. Oh well, life goes on and I'm excited about finally moving on.

Her friends called her a 'beautiful spirit'—always so upbeat and happy.

If you were Michelle's friend, you could expect to receive handwritten birthday cards and Christmas cards with Bible verses carefully chosen and neatly scribed on the left inside. Emails and handwritten letters were common—long, thoughtful pieces of prose filled with questions and personal information.

Michelle's emails to friends were always upbeat as she shared about her work and her visits to her family. She also wrote about some of her struggles to feel connected if she knew the recipient was also single. They would encourage each other in their singleness.

She wrote this of herself fifteen years prior to her death:

August 2002

I feel like I've always been the rock amongst my friends. The strong, dependable one, who is always there whenever they have a problem or just need to talk.

Michelle had a lot of best friends. Who wouldn't want a friend like her? She was fun to be around. She was willing and able to have the deep and meaningful conversations that made a difference. And she brought her contagious laugh and joy into each room she inhabited.

February 2013

I'm committed to being more thoughtful this year.

My goal this year is not to forget anyone's birthday. I know how blessed I feel when I receive a card in the mail, so I want to encourage others.

Amongst Michelle's friends were the kinds of people the Bible talks of. They were people others didn't always embrace and cherish; people who needed an encouraging friend and people who had low self-esteem.

Each person has a bucket that needs filling. If love is shown to us in the language we best receive it, our bucket fills up. We also fill our bucket by pursuing activities we enjoy and doing the jobs or hobbies God made us for.

Michelle's bucket was leaking faster than she or others could fill it. Even though she delighted in helping friends and clients, her deepest needs were not being met.

She tended to pull away from family members and friends when they married.

January 2015

My friend got engaged! I was probably a little surprised at my reaction, perhaps it was the finality of the situation that caused me to feel teary and in some ways grieve the loss of my closest friend and confidante. I have no doubt she will continue to try and still be my close friend but it will never be the same. I guess I also started to question again why my life has turned out the way it has and the challenges of being alone (obviously I still haven't learnt to be content in all circumstances!)

She felt the relationship with her female friends couldn't remain the same, distance ensued, and she sought new friendships.

Michelle was still a loyal friend, but she was inclined not to share as much with her wedded friends.

March 2013

My new friend from a nearby town is my latest confidante. We chat for hours which is lovely, thanks God.

Although she found a great sense of purpose in cheering others up and coming alongside them in their hour of need, it could be draining. Meanwhile, her own needs were being pushed further and further down.

Michelle wrote of one friend,

April 2013

I feel at present God's calling me to speak truth and hope into her life. I feel it is easy for us to focus on what we don't have, but I don't believe that is pleasing to God. He has provided an abundance for us and has huge destinies in store for His precious daughters. Tonight I'm encouraged to hold firm to that hope despite having no evidence to prove it. After all that's what faith is.

Michelle led Bible studies and prayer groups, and she led friends to the Lord. Her faithfulness in her own walk with Jesus was the foundation for her sharing this love with her friends. She bore much fruit as she connected with Jesus.[7]

November 2002

Never underestimate how much support the new Christian does need. Never forsake them.

July 2004

My friend came to life group and it was a great night. Everyone was very welcoming and we stayed late playing pool. On Thursday we girls caught up with another friend at Erina Fair and had a picnic at a park in Gosford. It was great.

'Well that was weird,' Michelle collapsed on the lounge.

Mum stirred the hot chocolate, teaspoon chinking against the warm mug. Her masseurs plodded on the wooden floorboards then she extended the beverage to my sister. 'What happened?'

'Somehow my pastor has convinced me to be the head of pastoral care at church now!'

Mum lowered herself on the recliner opposite and shook her head. 'I thought *you* wanted counselling. I thought you were scaling down with all the responsibility you have at work. I didn't think you wanted to take on anything else. You're helping enough people.'

Michelle sighed, sipping her hot drink. 'But I guess I'll do it, Mum. Somebody needs to.'

When in need of pastoral care herself, she became the head of her church's pastoral care team. This was not intentional on her part, but alas, she once again found herself giving more than she was receiving. But it wasn't easy to let others know of her deepest needs.

September 2014

It's so hard when people place expectations on you!

Throughout her life, Michelle held tight to the proverb, 'a real friend sticks closer than a brother.'[8] Jesus' friendship got Michelle through every season, and He held her hand to the end.

Five

Michelle the Counsellor

'What's going on, Nic?'

We were lolling on recliners nursing steamy mugs of hot chocolate and plunging our hands into a jar of mini Milky Ways and Snickers bars. My latest problem would come blurting out between bites of gooeyness.

'My friend has turned her back on me. I try hard to be thoughtful but somehow I've offended her.'

Michelle paused, slender fingers clasping her drink, her brown eyes searching mine. 'People suck, Dad,' she said with a soft laugh. It was one of our favourite movie quotes.[9] Even if I was crying, those words could make me smile.

Then wisdom rolled off her tongue, 'She sounds really immature. But Nic, you know you care too much about what people think.

25

'You can't change what happened, but you can control the way you think and feel about the situation. Let's pray about it.'

My journals are filled with moments in time when Michelle listened to me and prayed for me. She believed she was called to be a counsellor. *'I was born for this'* she wrote in her journals. And she was.

Michelle made people feel special. She loved the so-called 'unlovable'. Her beautiful spirit drew many to her side.

Arriving home in Australia after her first overseas trip, she began casual teaching. She was drawn to the 'behavioural' kids in her classrooms. Her heart of compassion bled for these children. She knew she had to pursue social work.

December 2010

The hardest question is how does one raise hope in a generation of disempowered, purposeless and goalless young people?

When she moved to Wagga Wagga with Lucinda for four years after returning from her working holiday to Canada, she began studying a social work degree and also worked in a juvenile detention centre. She loved her 'juvey' boys. She was determined to make a difference, one life at a time.

January 2011

I'm wondering if maybe God's calling me to some kind of prison ministry like Kairos? I want to help and support people whose loved ones are incarcerated.

With her full qualification in 2010, Michelle took a three-month Youth Justice position in North Queensland. She worked as an OOHC (Out of Home Care) caseworker for DOCs[10] in northern New South Wales. Next, she headed back to the country town where our parents reside to work as a case manager for children and families through The Benevolent Society—Brighter Futures. And finally, she obtained her most treasured position as child protection counsellor for NSW Health.

March 2011

My gift of counselling was confirmed so much more as I got chatting with two girls. Sometimes I feel like as long as I'm listening to others' problems and helping them, I won't have to be exposed myself. I feel I have huge insecurities. But God says, 'I have called you to be a healer of the mind and as such I am healing you of your weaknesses so you can stand in for others.'

Michelle always had a way with children. Her first degree was a Bachelor of Education (Early Childhood). She was always great in caring for children in daycare and school, as well as loving her nieces and nephews.

I can only imagine the warmth and love Michelle gave to her clients as she met with them in their homes in her role as child protection counsellor. How she championed the children and gave hope and wise professional advice to the parents. What a difference she must have made to the families in her town.

Michelle became a White Ribbon ambassador, known in her community for this role as she organised events and was the face of these special days. White Ribbon Australia advocates against men's violence against women.[11]

June 2015

Yesterday I attended the White Ribbon event at the Rugby Club. It was fantastic to see so many people there.

Michelle stayed faithfully working in her child protection counselling role whilst her team changed staff time after time. Meanwhile, her supervisor stated that she was miles ahead of her colleagues in terms of workload.

Not only did she bear the load of her clients' lives, she also sought to support and encourage her workmates. And there was tension in the work environment.

May 2010

My job is proving to be very tiring. I'm travelling one and a half hours a day to and from work.

February 2011

It's been an absolutely crazy week. I felt so exhausted last night.

April 2015

This week I've really struggled; not wanting to get out of bed and just feeling really down.

August 2016

The new draft guidelines in many respects are not workable. I'm quite concerned with what my role will look like in the future.

At times Michelle reached out when she was feeling overwhelmed. One time, after writing in her journal, she met with some church friends for prayer. She had written, *I can't help it, I feel completely abandoned! I can't shake the feeling that everyone's lives are moving on except mine. What a week!'*

Michelle had a fear of being alone. Her church friends prayed for her, assuring her that God had not forgotten her, and gave her the following Bible verses from the book of Isaiah;

'Pay attention, O Jacob, for you are my servant, O Israel. I, the Lord, made you, and I will not forget you. I have swept away your sins like a cloud. I have scattered your offenses like the morning mist. Oh, return to me, for I have paid the price to set you free.'[12]

Michelle was an avid journal writer and, over time, her journals contain the ups and downs of her life, and the depression and anxiety she tended to spiral into. She was moody. But until 2017, she managed to cope through the bouts of hidden mental illness.

Six

Heartbroken Michelle

The pain. How long it's been there I cannot tell and yet I feel I've endured it for years. It's more intense now, though. The throbbing ache resounding throughout my chest causes me to bring my fingertips gingerly to my heart. I casually look down and am shocked to see the small red droplets clashing starkly against my tan fingers. On closer inspection, I view the wound. The slit is small, yet drop after drop of my precious life's blood relentlessly flows.

I panic! Rushing to the cupboard, I fumble clumsily through ointment, Band-Aids and creams until I find a thin bandage. I place it gently over the wound, attaching it there permanently with tape.

Life goes on. Soon I forget the pain; I grow desensitized to it and yet it's always there. I change the bandage every now and again when the blood has soaked through it, but I think nothing of it.

The dressing is as much a part of me now as eating and sleeping.

Yet I am pedantic about not letting others see my pain. I spend as much time ensuring this as I do treating my wound. Why do I care so much? I'm embarrassed. I'm not sure I could endure my greatest fear being exposed. It's survival of the fittest. Not that I believe I will be hunted down and viciously murdered, but isn't being looked at patronisingly a far worse fate?

I go on pretending. I like my chances better this way. I pretend until I sense something is wrong. The pain, it's sharper, more intense. I peel back the bandage to view the wound. It's worse. The blood bubbles up from deep within and spills out the festering gash.

I'm surprised and yet I continue to apply another clean white bandage. The quick fix solution is far more appealing than any other alternate answer. I comprehend the severity of the injury and know that it could lead to hospitalisation, possibly even death, and yet I continue to ignore it.

It's increasingly harder to function. My mind is constantly consumed with my problem, my pain, to such a degree that I can no longer comprehend the pain of others. I'm like a machine, going about my appointed duties in life with no feeling, while I close myself off from those around me.

How long can I last? Is there hope for me?

... I pretend to be happy, that it doesn't bother me and I'm a very good actress. Meanwhile something's dying.

I begin to lose hope, lose faith. I go through bouts of depression. One minute I'm on top of the world; the next I'm in the pits of hell.

Michelle wrote this vivid imagery for a book we envisaged, 'Single ... But Not Satisfied'. Working together we created chapters about singleness—how we felt being single in our early twenties, and how disappointed we were with life, with church, with dashed hopes and dreams.

I see clues in this piece by Michelle. She was hurting. She was lonely. And she wanted to hide the pain.

Hiding when hurting.

Mum remembers when Michelle received her school certificate results at the end of year ten (aged fifteen). She threw the papers straight in the bin and she ran and hid in her wardrobe. Michelle chose to hide when she was hurting.

I think this is significant. When she was hurting emotionally, Michelle hid. She hid her feelings. She hid her pain.

'So Nic,' Michelle cleared her throat and tapped her fingernail against the pepper shaker. We were sitting in a local service station diner finishing off our hamburgers and hot chips. 'I've got something to tell you.'

I swallowed my beef and beetroot and reached for my glass of water. 'Yeah?'

'Remember Ashton from spring camp in Canada?'

'Yeah.'

Michelle took a slow breath. She turned the pepper shaker around a couple of revolutions. 'Well, we've been emailing.'

She looked for my reaction and I know my eyes bulged.

My sister laughed a little, then stopped. 'Crazy, hey? I really liked him ... Anyway, it's all over now. He doesn't feel the same way about me.

'Not to mention we live in different countries.'

She answered my many questions and I remember my mind struggling to comprehend how she could keep secrets and 'go it alone'. The communication between her and Ashton had been going on for weeks. Yet she hadn't told a soul.

It was this evening at the diner that I recalled after she divulged her next two heartbreaks concerning men. Again the secrecy. Again the silence.

Michelle had always been close to her family, but she wasn't willing to share the journey of her crushes and her romance and her heartbreak … until relationships ended. We all face heartbreak. It's part of the human condition. But facing it alone is devastating.

According to Wesley Lifeforce Suicide Prevention Training, there are precipitating and escalating factors that can lead to suicide.

1. Experience of loss
2. Experience of crisis
3. Trigger event or tipping point
4. Suicidal thoughts and behaviour[13]

This experience of loss includes all the disappointments in life that pile up one after another until there is a mountain of them.

For Michelle, I believe she experienced loss each time a sister or close friend wed. Although she was my maid of honour, she was somewhat distant in the days around my marriage. In hindsight, I think she was trying to cope with her grief, and she poured it all into her new puppy.

He was sick before my big day, and he ended up dying. Michelle's focus was on her puppy and she pushed down how she felt about 'losing' me.

Conversations Michelle had with Mum and me told us she experienced loss in the times when she felt rejected by men. She lost physical health as she was diagnosed with kidney cancer and endometriosis. She lost her freedom. She felt she would lose her job. She lost the hope of ever having children of her own. And finally, she lost her mental health.

At this point, she had experienced crisis and reached her tipping point. Throw in a lack of sleep and loss of appetite, and it was a slide into hopelessness. She had slid this way many years before, but not this deep or this far.

April 2012

My depression has worried me this time. I haven't had particular suicidal thoughts (as in a plan) but my mind has definitely been wandering into that territory, God help me. I do just want the pain and discomfort to end so badly.

Michelle took things hard, like losing in a board game or losing a set of tennis, or not receiving a book or certificate at speech night at the end of a school year. The big feelings would overtake her and she would run off in a rage, tears streaming down her face.

We called it melancholy. Her heart called it loss.

Seven

Michelle's Last Months

Two years before her suicide, Michelle faced a setback and, for about five days, she could barely eat, sleep or function. *I have never experienced anything like this in my entire life and it has been terrifying!'* She described her set back as 'soul crushing'.

A series of disappointments with friendships and relationships affected her hope for the future. She took incidents personally, and it's possible she had undiagnosed PTSD (Post-Traumatic Stress Disorder) from the shock and trauma in her personal life as well as her working life.

Six months before the suicide, Michelle had trouble sleeping again. She'd been considering changing jobs within her field. This led her to participate in JIRT (Joint Investigation Response Team) training.

The traumatic, brutal images Michelle had to view as part of this training impacted her heart.

Michelle's health was of concern to her as well. She had an operation the year before she died, and, in June of the year she died, she was scheduled to have another. The specialist had found cancer in her right kidney.

I drove home from my appointment through a ferocious lightning storm and just prayed for protection, at one point barely missing a tree that had been struck by lightning. The roads were wet and my mind in turmoil.

All of this was weighing heavily on her heart. Anxiety caused her to jump to conclusions, engage in forward-thinking and slip into despair. The stronger these thoughts and feelings became, the more she threw herself into work and the community. Busyness kept her going. She would find the next person who needed help and comfort, all the while pushing her own needs and fears further down.

So with the kidney operation scheduled, she did what she always loved doing—she took a road trip. As I've read Michelle's journals and reflected on her last months, I don't believe she intended her road trip as a way of saying goodbye to her friends, but I know it looked that way in hindsight. I think it was more about doing something she found fun, something that usually lifted her spirits, before having to 'face the music' and go through with the operation she didn't want to have. Sadly, the trip took a big emotional toll on her. She was grief-stricken, telling friends of her diagnosis, and discouraged by one particular response she received before she returned home.

In the back of her mind, I think she worried that cancer or another physical illness may one day take her life. But I don't think she had a long-term plan to end her own life.

Yesterday I returned to the doctor to receive the results of my renal ultrasound. It appears the cyst on my left kidney has grown. The doctor also said, 'Cancerous cysts present this way.' I'm thankful I have everything covered should the worst happen. I know this sounds morbid and fatalistic but when you hear 'cancer' it's hard not to think that way.

As her sister, the first I knew that Michelle's mental health was in crisis was eleven days before her death. Our parents were supposed to be coming to my home for my son's birthday party on the weekend of 13–14th May. It was the Friday when Mum phoned me, sounding out of breath.

'Michelle's not coping. She's not sleeping or eating, and she's having trouble making decisions. I'm sorry, Nicki. We won't be coming over this weekend. I've got to stay here and look after your sister.'

It was Mother's Day in Australia, Sunday 14th May, when Michelle presented at emergency at her local hospital. To be hospitalised in the town where she worked as a child protection counsellor was both embarrassing and shameful to her. She was petrified of being seen by her clients or workmates. Having helped so many local families battling with mental health and domestic violence, she didn't want to look as though she was unfit in her own mind. She worked in health but felt the need to go out of the area to be treated.

Our parents brought her over to my city on the Tuesday. She was not admitted to the mental health ward. Dad,

Mum and Michelle spent the night at my place. Little did I know it was the last time I would ever see my sister.

When I found out she was awake at about four am, and my husband was out working the night shift, Michelle and I talked for over an hour. Not knowing she was suicidal and not trained in mental health first aid, I didn't ask the pertinent questions. We talked for over an hour. I knew she was feeling the pressure of her finances and not being able to work.

'You have cared for countless people in your life. You need to let people care for you now. You are not super-woman.' I said, hoping she would feel comforted.

I regret heading to work because, as I was leaving, I could see and sense she was getting anxious. If I hadn't gone to teach that day, could I have stopped her from dying? Could I have arranged help for her in my city, where she could have stayed with me? Endless questions with no answers and no chance to turn back time.

There were four hospitals involved in Michelle's case. After failing to be admitted to two, she hyperventilated on the way home the next day and Dad and Mum took her to another base hospital. This hospital diagnosed a high risk of suicide.

She rested in the safe room overnight, with constant observation by a guard standing at her door. This hospital is required to send patients on to another different hospital, so she was unable to return to the hospital in my city. The staff there decided not to hold her overnight. A few days later, Michelle's life was over.

Dead.

Too young.

A life lost too soon.

Michelle's mind had started to cave in with the weight of everything wrong in her life and the lives of her clients upon her. She wanted to fix herself and make herself better. She didn't seek help until things were desperate, and our parents had to seek help for her.

I penned in my journal,

'I love you, Michelle. I know nothing can bring you back and you were really suffering. I forgive you for taking your own life. I know the pain. I only wish I could have had more time to walk with you through this wilderness. See you in heaven. Love always and forever, Nicki xx'

Eight

How to Help a Loved One Who Is Suicidal

I'm coming from a place of lived experience as one who has been bereaved by suicide and faced my own mental illness and suicidal ideation.[14] I'm not an expert in this field. I have completed a one-day training course with Wesley Lifeforce on Suicide Prevention. I've also completed a two-day Mental Health First Aid training course and I have attended the National Suicide Prevention Conference in Australia.

There are plenty of myths surrounding suicide. Attending a Suicide Prevention Training course is one of the best ways to gain understanding and the most up-to-date information and terminology surrounding suicide.

Importantly, we now say a person suicided or died by suicide, rather than committed suicide.

The term 'committed' came from decades ago when suicide was seen as a crime, a sin, and a person was 'committed' to an asylum.

Stigmatised terminology includes: successful suicide, completed suicide, failed attempt at suicide and unsuccessful suicide. These terms need to be removed from our vocabularies. Appropriate terminology to date is ended his/her life, non-fatal attempt at suicide and attempt to end his/her life.

The reason people suicide is multifactorial. 'The causes appear to be a complex mix of life events, social, geographical, cultural, family and socio-economic factors combined with genetic makeup, mental and physical health support from family, friends and the ability to manage life events and bounce back from adversity.'[15]

Suicidal ideation can ebb and flow, depending on circumstances. A person may be depressed and isolated, lacking self-worth and purpose. They may be taking illegal drugs or abusing alcohol. A person may feel they don't belong and they've lost hope.

American clinical psychologist Edwin S Schneidman first came up with the term 'psychache' to describe 'intense emotional and psychological pain that eventually becomes intolerable and which cannot be abated by means that were previously successful—as the primary motivation for suicide'.[16]

Even the best psychologist doesn't know when a person is threatening suicide that night or actually going to follow through. Psychache is different for each individual. It's a crisis of their deepest sense of self.

As friends and family members of loved ones who are facing mental illness, we can feel powerless to help. Some of our excuses include: 'What if I try to help and they do it anyway?', 'I don't know what to do or say' or 'I am not a trained professional'.

The good news is there's something we can do. The S.A.L.T. strategy can help prevent suicide.

S—See the warning signs

A—Ask about suicide intent

L—Listen to the person

T—Tell or TAKE the person to appropriate help

As previously mentioned, the precipitating events and escalating factors include experience of loss, experience of crisis, trigger event or tipping point, suicidal thoughts and behaviour.

Being a good listener is key to helping someone who is feeling suicidal. By listening, we bear witness to a person's pain. Reflective listening validates their emotions, reflecting on what the person is feeling rather than reflecting on their situation. Is your loved one saying, 'I'm going to kill myself', 'It's all too hard' or 'I'm just a burden to everyone'? Hear what they are saying.

Watch for dramatic changes in mood—either feeling euphoric or withdrawing further. Are they putting their affairs in order?

Discover what the person may have experienced or lost. Remember, it's not your job to fix the suicidality that has come on over weeks, months or years. Your intervention is to get them professional help.

One of the key concerns we have as a nation is that by asking someone if they're planning to suicide, we'll put ideas in their head. The research says this is not the case.

So it's time to be direct. Ask, 'Are you thinking of killing yourself?', 'Are you thinking about ending your life?' or 'Are you thinking about suicide?'

If your loved one admits that they are thinking these things, listen and normalise. Say, 'It's not uncommon for people who have ... (fill in the blank) ... to think of taking their own life.'

Since you have discovered what your loved one may have lost, identify the losses. Ask, 'Have you thought about how you might end your life?' Also ask if they have the means to end their life.

- Take them to professional help
- You can help keep the person safe by finding layers of support for them
- Stay overnight at their place or have them at your place
- Book a long appointment with their GP
- Call the Mental Health Access Line or Lifeline[17]
- Head to Emergency at your local hospital

There are more and more organisations rising up in our communities to help in both crisis times and times where ongoing support is needed.

If you're like me, someone who has already been bereaved by suicide, I'm so sorry. Know that you have not failed. You aren't responsible.

You did your best with what you knew at the time, and you deserve a big hug and a cup of tea.

It's not easy living with this kind of grief. The Precious Michelle community exists to encourage you and point you to professional help as well. Carers and grievers alike need support. Set aside ten to thirty minutes every day to do something kind for yourself.

It's a hard road. Let's walk it together, one step at a time.

Hope for Your Hurting Heart

On my way back to the country town where are parents reside for Michelle's funeral, I read through a gift book I was about to give to my father, 'Letter to a Grieving Heart' by Billy Sprague. Sprague faced the death of his fiancée, a beloved grandmother and also a favourite college professor.

I trusted this author because I knew he knew the depth of grief I was facing. They say suicide grief is different from any other form of grief, but Billy knew a similar pain.

He wrote, 'I am sorry you have to face life with this kind of wound.'[18]

'No one can talk away the pain. Grief drains most words of their power anyway.'[19]

He also wrote that his friend walked right into the agony with him. That's what friends do. And what was most helpful to him was the practical stuff—his friend doing dishes, restocking the refrigerator, paying bills, answering the phone, lighting a fire in his fireplace, making him something warm to drink, reading the Psalms, bringing him a pot of homemade soup.

Billy's friend prayed over him, 'Dear Lord, don't let Billy's memories remain anchors that he has to drag along. Turn them to treasures he can carry with him.'[20]

I'm sorry you have to face life with this kind of wound. I wish you didn't. I wish time could be turned back and events altered. But it can't, and we're left because our loved one's gone.

Sometimes it is best to sit with the pain and go gently. Don't allow the passing of time to guilt you into feeling worse or thinking that you should be getting on with your life and letting go.

I was in shock when I heard the news that my sister had died. I was told when I was teaching my class at primary school. The office manager and the school chaplain knocked on the door of my classroom. I knew something was wrong.

'Do you have your phone, Nicki?' the office manager asked.

As I exited the classroom and the chaplain sat in my place, the office manager said, 'Can you please phone your father?'

I whispered, 'It's bad news?'

She nodded.

I could barely believe it when my Dad said, 'Nicki, Michelle is in the arms of Jesus.'

I'm writing this nearly three years after the event and tears are stinging the corners of my eyes. I have that feeling in my nose, that tingling where your mind reminds you of the overwhelming emotions that swirled within you that fateful day.

'But I just spoke to her this morning. She sounded really good ...' my words trailed off as I contemplated what had happened. It was unbelievable. I was cold. I needed to sit down. I could feel the colour drain from my face.

I'd been worried about Michelle for the past eleven days. And now, more than ever, her pain was mine. They say suicide doesn't end the pain—it passes it to the surviving relatives. Even so, I didn't blame Michelle. I felt sad—for her, for me and for my family.

I wished Michelle had been kept safe in hospital, but I was told that even hospitals can't always keep patients one hundred percent safe. I wished Michelle could have held on until things started to improve. But she couldn't.

Deep breath.

I saw my psychologist—the beautiful grandmotherly-type figure who had seen me at my worst, as I was heading for psychotic depression. Her words were a healing balm to my fragile soul. She stressed the importance of self-care in the days of grief.

- Have a massage
- Have a bubble bath with candles
- Go to nature (for me, the beach)
- Make an extra psychologist appointment
- See friends
- Listen to music

- Ask someone to have the kids so you can look after you

When feelings arise in dreams, they want to get out. Even in the daytime, when you feel certain things, you need to go softly. Do what is needed. Ask for a hug. Take a walk. Listen to music. It's not just distraction, it's dealing with grief.

When people start talking to you about their problems in this time of grief, it's okay to politely ask them to talk to you about it some other time. It's also fine not to answer calls or to write back that you're having a quiet week.

Like a baby needs to be held by somebody, you need to be held and nurtured at this time, and not just by people hugging you.

My psychologist spoke into my life concerning my unique family and the choices Michelle made. And it helped. I saw her a few times in those initial months of grief. I still see her when I need to. Even psychologists see psychologists! We all need someone who is there for us for that hour session. It's all about us and it's a way we self-care and process events and feelings with a trained professional who cares and with whom we have a rapport.

Because I am a Christian, I also sought out further prayer ministry. I had previously had VMTC (Victorious Ministries Through Christ) prayer ministry and had attended a VMTC training school.

This was helpful to me because I had a soul tie to Michelle. We had been two peas in a pod for much of our lives.

Even though we were sisters, there was a soul tie like a marriage relationship.

It was a great session where I forgave and received healing spiritually.

Some Bible verses that were given to me at that time were:

From Isaiah, 'Then your salvation will come like the dawn, and your wounds will quickly heal. Your godliness will lead you forward, and the glory of the Lord will protect you from behind.'[21]

From Matthew, 'God blesses those who mourn, for they will be comforted.'[22]

The greatest hope I drew from my initial season of grief was that God is in control, Michelle was in heaven and Jesus was with me. I believe God walks with us through every season of our lives and He is with us when we find ourselves in the darkest depths.

If you'd like to learn more about my Christian faith, please head to my website or message me via social media. I'd love to share with you the reasons for the hope I have.

Ten

Letter to Michelle

'Dear Michelle,

Hi.

Well, we are approaching the second of your birthdays without you here on Earth. I realised I have not penned you a letter since you've been gone. I haven't been able to talk to you for a couple of years. It feels good to be able to write you a letter. To write your name.

Where to start?

The trigger for writing this letter was an article I read in the Facebook community—LOSS Loved Ones Suicide Survivors support group. A woman had lost her brother to suicide fifteen years before, when he was twenty-one and she was twenty-four. She mentioned writing letters to him.

I've been thinking about writing your story and calling the book, Precious Michelle. I realised to do that, I kind of need to consult with you. And I need to process my own feelings. And whilst I'll never 'get over' your sudden death, I think I need to come to the right place within my head and heart in order to write the book.

Will you write this book with me? Can we take this journey together? Because I really want the words to reflect your heart, and what you would want the world to know about you and your story.

I know you can't whisper in my ear or tell me in so many words. But I know our mutual best friend, Jesus Christ, can do that for us because He knows both of us. He knows the journey. His Holy Spirit can give me the revelation.

I know you didn't aspire to be famous. You weren't a 'limelight' person. But your light shone so brightly and touched so many hearts and lives. And your journals are filled with insights and beautiful dreams and visions from His heart. So with you at the forefront of my mind and heart, I'm going to do this. With respect for you and knowing I'll see you again and be accountable to God, I write and speak.

Just as you needed to counsel people, I need to write and speak. We are His mouthpiece. Like Aaron did for Moses in the Bible, I will do for you. 'Aaron will be your spokesman to the people. He will be your mouthpiece, and you will stand in the place of God for him, telling him what to say.'[23]

We were two halves, two peas in a pod. We were different, with unique callings.

I love you, Michelle.

Until we meet again ...

Love, Nicki x'

Afterword

A Note About Suicide and the Christian

You've probably heard of and possibly believed that people who suicide go to hell. I don't believe that is true for the born-again Christian and this is why.

Heaven is the eternal address for people who trust in Jesus for their salvation, living their lives walking with Him. If a Christian suffers from a mental illness for weeks, months or years, and they make a decision in one of their moments of irrational thinking to end their life, they are still saved. Their salvation is not in jeopardy because, at one point, they lost hope and succumbed to the most drastic and devastating effects of this illness.

A friend put it to me like this, 'If you were a Christian and accidentally fell to your death from a rooftop, swearing on the way down, would you go to hell? No. Jesus' death covers your sins past, present and future.

And although the Bible warns against wilfully sinning because you are saved by grace, this sin does not keep you from heaven.'

Is suicide a sin? Is it the unforgivable sin? The only unforgivable sin I read in the Bible is the sin of blaspheming the Holy Spirit. To blaspheme the Holy Spirit is to reject the salvation that God has provided for us in His Son.

Having said this, I am not a proponent of suicide.

I believe anyone who dies without Christ will spend eternity without Him. Being suicidal is a hopeless state of existence, yet there is a way out. Being a Christian may not protect you from suicidal ideation, mental illness or taking your own life, but Jesus is with you in your anguish.

I don't believe suicide is the way God wants anybody to die. Jesus came to bring life, and life in abundance.

If your loved one is a Christian and they're battling with mental illness and suicidal ideation, they need cognitive help. Praying for them and reading the Bible to them are great things to do, and there is a spiritual war raging. But to think these disciplines are the sole answer to becoming well from this illness is a fallacy.

It's my prayer that, as a society, we don't lose any more precious souls to suicide. It's time to speak up, tell our stories and engage in suicide prevention.

The Bible says, 'For I know the plans I have for you,' says the Lord. 'They are plans for good and not for disaster, to give you a future and a hope.'[24]

Michelle's Vision

On 23rd December 2016, Michelle wrote in her journal, *'I feel 2017 will be extremely significant.'*

I'm sure she didn't know she would die in 2017. But in 2017, she was set free from her pain in this world.

Michelle is gone, but her legacy remains, and it's not without impact. As you read this beautiful vision God gave her, be encouraged. The spiritual realm is real. Jesus is alive. And He wants you to come into His Kingdom at the end of your earthly life.

I saw myself dressed in a beautiful golden gown which shone like silk and was covered in sequins. I was standing with a group of believers. They were dressed the same and we were praising God with our hands raised.

All of a sudden God showed me a magnificent crown and we all became gems within the crown.

If the *Precious Michelle* documentary or book touches your life in any way, we would love to hear from you. Head to https://www.nickijeffery.com or find us on social media. On Facebook: Nicki Jeffery author or Precious Michelle. On Instagram: search for @suicidepreventionaustralia.

Notes

PREFACE

1   Excerpt from one of Michelle's journals.

2   There has been extensive work undertaken to improve the culture and practice of the hospitals concerned and serious HR implications arose. I would not like to negatively impact on this positive work and potentially create further staff distress.

MICHELLE THE SISTER

3   'Saturday Disney' is a long running Australian children's television program which aired on the Seven Network in Australia for over 26 years, with the first episode going to air on 27 January 1990.

4   'DuckTales' is an American animated television series, produced by Walt Disney Television Animation and distributed by Buena Vista Television. 'TaleSpin' is an American animated television series first aired in 1990 as a preview on Disney Channel and later that year as part of The Disney Afternoon. 'Saved by the Bell' is an American television sitcom which was broadcast by NBC from August 20, 1989 to May 22, 1993.

MICHELLE THE TRAVELLER

5   Psalm 2:8.

6   Excerpt from 'Faith-based Travels: A Devotional Guidebook for the Faith-filled Traveller', by Nicki Jeffery (2015). Ark House Press. Mona Vale. Australia. Pages 202, 203.

MICHELLE THE FRIEND

7   In John 15, the Bible talks about Jesus being the vine and we the branches. Michelle was connected to Him and she bore much fruit for the Kingdom.

8   Proverbs 18:24.

MICHELLE THE COUNSELLOR

9   '10 Things I Hate About You', Touchstone Pictures, 1999.

10   DOCS stands for Department of Community Services. DOCS has been renamed FACS, which stands for Family and Community Services.

11   White Ribbon Australia, accessed 23rd January 2020
        https://www.whiteribbon.org.au/

12   Isaiah 44:21,22.

HEARTBROKEN MICHELLE

13   Wesley LifeForce Suicide Prevention Training workshop workbook, Carlingford, NSW, 2018.

HOW TO HELP A LOVED ONE WHO IS SUICIDAL

14   Suicidal ideation refers to thinking about or planning suicide.

15   Wesley LifeForce Suicide Prevention Training workshop workbook, Carlingford NSW, 2018.

16   Shneidman, E.S., 'Suicide as Psychache: A Clinical Approach to Self-Destructive Behavior'. Northvale, NJ/London: Jason Aronson, Inc., p258, 1993.

17   NSW Mental Health Access Line 1800 011 511. Lifeline 13 11 14.

HOPE FOR YOUR HURTING HEART

18   Sprague, B., 'Letter to a Grieving Heart: Comfort and Hope for those who hurt'. Eugene, OR/ USA: Harvest House Publishers, p5, 2001.

19   Sprague, B., 'Letter to a Grieving Heart: Comfort and Hope for those who hurt'. Eugene, OR/ USA: Harvest House Publishers, p6, 2001.

20   Sprague, B., 'Letter to a Grieving Heart: Comfort and Hope for those who hurt'. Eugene, OR/ USA: Harvest House Publishers, p52, 2001.

21   Isaiah 58:8.

22   Matthew 5:4.

LETTER TO MICHELLE

23   Exodus 4:16.

AFTERWORD

24   Jeremiah 29:11.

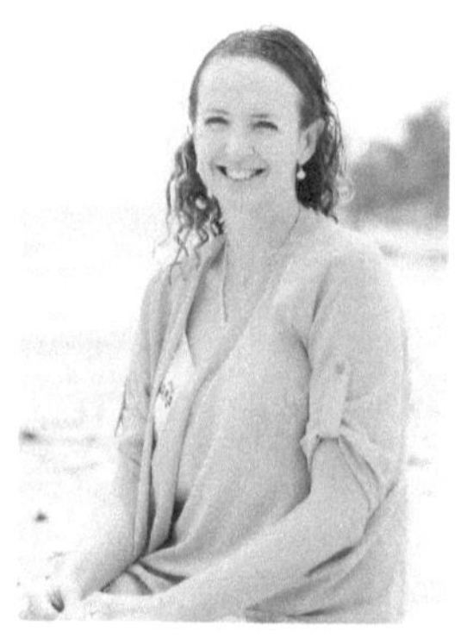

About the Author

Nicki Jeffery grew up on a sheep and wheat farm in central New South Wales, Australia. She graduated from university with a Bachelor of Education and enjoys primary school teaching. Nicki loves to encourage and inspire, and *Precious Michelle* is her third non-fiction book. She lives on the mid north coast with her husband Nathan, their sons Matthew and Ethan, their puppy Jessie, their cat Gracie and two important chooks Strawberry and Joy.

You can connect with me on:

🌐 https://www.nickijeffery.com

🐦 https://twitter.com/nicki_jeffery

f https://www.facebook.com/Precious-Michelle-101169008065046

Subscribe to my newsletter:

✉ https://www.nickijeffery.com/blog

Also by Nicki Jeffery

Sisters Nicki and Michelle fulfilled their childhood dream to travel to Canada and the States on working holiday visas when they were in their twenties, which provided the inspiration for *Faith-based Travels: A Devotional Guidebook for the Faith-filled Traveller.* In her thirties, Nicki battled post-natal depression and psychosis in the early years of her sons' lives. She wrote *Encouraging Mums with Hope: Light in the Darkness of Maternal Depression* to empower women of faith during this season. Sadly, Michelle died by suicide in 2017. *Precious Michelle: A Sister Reminisces a Life Lost to Suicide* is a personal account of a beautiful, bubbly woman of God who lost her life to mental illness, yet inspired many in her 36 years to live for Jesus.

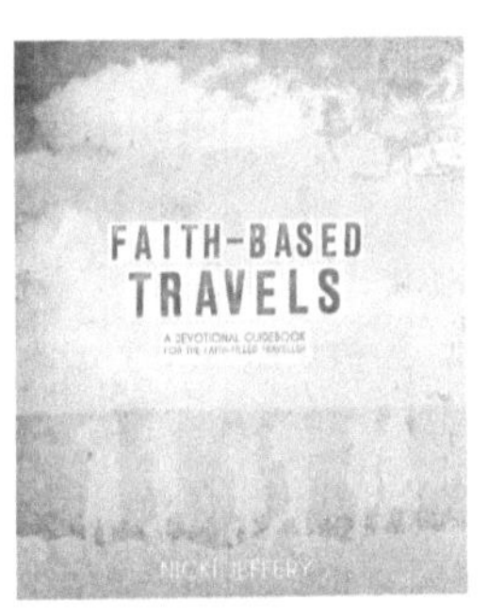

Faith-based Travels: A Devotional Guidebook for the Faith-filled Traveller

What kind of traveller are you?

In search of adventure, seeking new experiences, hoping to improve a language, aspiring to work and holiday, a missionary or vagrant sojourner?

No matter what your flavour, *Faith-based Travels* is a spiritual tool for experiencing the world as a Christian traveller. This devotional delves into the realities of living out of a suitcase, from backpacker hostels to home stays.

The author, a traveller herself, will take you on a journey from planning a trip overseas, to living it out, returning home and reconnecting in the community. Each devotion concludes with thought-provoking questions and a prayer.

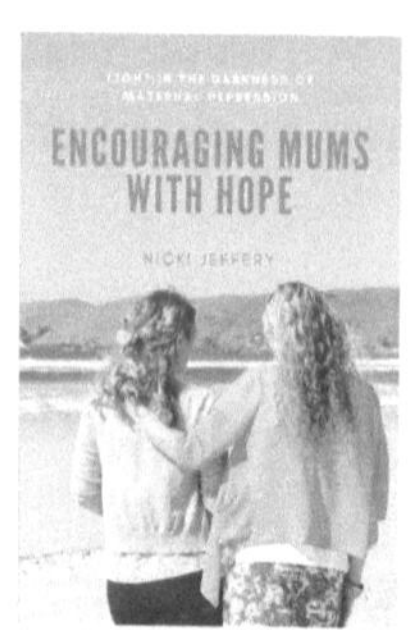

Encouraging Mums with Hope: Light in the Darkness of Maternal Depression

Are you a mother struggling to cope?

Are you constantly overwhelmed and anxious?

Do you long for better mental health to be able to care for yourself and your family?

When storms engulf you and everything is dismal and grey, *Encouraging Mums With Hope: Light in the Darkness of Maternal Depression* will bring you back into the sunshine.

Australian author Nicki Jeffery and a large group of mothers, health professionals and pastoral care workers address BODY, SOUL, and SPIRIT in this uplifting book.

Filled with tips, practical strategies, and loads of encouragement, you will discover that you are not alone.

www.ingramcontent.com/pod-product-compliance
Lightning Source LLC
Chambersburg PA
CBHW030826060726
47590CB00004B/1413